Strength Training For Fat Loss:

Workouts, Exercises and Diet Tips For Effective Weight Loss

By

Charles Maldonado

Table of Contents

Introduction 5

Chapter 1. The Basic Principles of Strength Training For Fat Loss 7

Chapter 2. Foods You Need to Eat For Strength Training and Fat Loss... 10

Chapter 3. Strength Training Exercises 14

Chapter 4. Training Plan... 17

    For The Cardio.. 17

    Workout 20

    Workout A: Full Body 23

    Workout B: Full Body 28

    Reminders 34

Conclusion... 36

Thank You Page 37

Strength Training For Fat Loss: Workouts, Exercises and Diet Tips For Effective Weight Loss

By Charles Maldonado

© Copyright 2015 Charles Maldonado

Reproduction or translation of any part of this work beyond that permitted by section 107 or 108 of the 1976 United States Copyright Act without permission of the copyright owner is unlawful. Requests for permission or further information should be addressed to the author.

This publication is designed to provide accurate and authoritative information in regard to the subject matter covered. This work is sold with the understanding that the publisher is not engaged in rendering legal, accounting, or other professional services. If legal advice or other expert assistance is required, the services of a competent professional person should be sought.

First Published, 2015

Printed in the United States of America

Introduction

Strength training is being done to enhance metabolic rate, overall body shape, and of course it has weight loss benefits. When people engage in strength training exercises, it's not just about pushing your body to the limit and lifting weight, but it's also about changing the diet, lifestyle, routine, weekly goal, and determination to achieve a better body. For some people who don't have any idea about strength training, they cannot be blamed for having some common misconception about strength training and that's what this book is for.

They will be informed about the principles of strength training to lose fat, what foods they should eat, what strength training exercises they can do, how many days are required to achieve the best results, how training days should look like, and what kind of training plan needs to be followed. Having a training plan helps the person not to get confused about what to do the next day and how long they should train. All of the facts found in this book are based on research and it has been proven to be effective for strength training. If you are currently doing any kind of exercise, you will be able to compare what makes strength training different when you try to do the exercises for strength training, but you must be assisted by a trainer when doing them so you can have more support and you can be told if you are doing it correctly or not especially when it comes to proper form because that can affect the effectiveness of the workout. If you decide to start strength training, you need to stay focused and dedicated because it requires hard work and self-discipline. There are some foods that you need to cut back on or stop eating completely especially if it's bad for your health. You need to be in good condition when performing exercises so that you will be able to execute them well and have the results that you really want.

After you have read this book, you will know where to start, what to do, and better understand the principles behind strength training.

Chapter 1. The Basic Principles of Strength Training For Fat Loss

Start with your meals

You need to change the way you eat because if you are used to eating excessive amounts of food that will greatly affect the results of your strength training and also your overall health. In any exercise or workout regimen, this is very important this can principle can be applied to any of them. You can imagine dividing your plate into four parts –one part should be for the lean protein, another part for the healthy carbohydrates like whole grain bread and brown rice, and fill up the 2 remaining parts with vegetables.

Get on your feet

Do not make sudden changes in your workout routine because it can cause injury, soreness, and you will become overwhelmed. What you must do is to walk more every day which is already a form of light cardio and will help burn a few extra calories in a day to help you with the results. Workouts don't have to be hard for you to see the results and little activities add up over time so you can get the results that you desire.

Lift more

Lifting weights added into your routine will be good for your overall health. Your metabolic rate will increase, and you will burn more calories every day. You will also have the benefit of gaining better looking muscles that are toned and more defined. Eat protein and carbohydrates before your workout and after your workout for recovery. You will see results better because you allow your body to recover.

Your snacks should be more protein-based

You will surely get hungry from time to time and avoid snacks that are high in sugar, fat, and carbohydrates which can affect the results that you want to get. A cereal bar is a common choice, but it does not really contain any of the important components that you need which will only lead you to eat more, but without getting the nutrients that you really need. You need to pick snacks that are packed with protein because it benefits your metabolism and overall fat loss.

Get enough sleep

You should be getting enough sleep because lack of sleep leaves you with more food cravings and you will have the tendency to just eat what you can grab regardless if it's healthy or not. Lack of sleep also affects the way you perform workouts and your condition while exercising will also not be good.

Chapter 2. Foods You Need to Eat For Strength Training and Fat Loss

Eggs- Aside from the high protein content of eggs which is 7g, the yolk has the most nutrients because 3.5 g of protein is in there, you will also be getting vitamins a, d, e, and the cholesterol you need to so that your testosterone levels will increase. You should not worry about the yolk if you don't have bad cholesterol.

Fish oil – This helps in reducing inflammation of the skin and joints. This will also make your body become lower and the level of your testosterone will increase. The body needs 9000 mg of DHA in a day which you can get from fish oil supplement.

Wild salmon – This is a very good source of omega-3 fats which is important for the health and it is good for the heart. You will get 20 g of omega-3 for every 100 g of wild salmon.

Berries – These contain a lot of antioxidants especially raspberries. Antioxidants are good for helping prevent cancer, diseases in the eyes and heart. It is also good to eat fresh berries with oatmeal.

Yogurt – This contains bacteria that are good for your gastrointestinal health. You need to get the plain yogurt because yogurts being sold in stores that have fruits contain a lot of sugar. You can also eat this with flax seeds and berries.

Extra virgin olive oil – This contains 70% of the monounsaturated fat that helps your body against cancer and heart diseases.

Broccoli – This has phytochemicals that fights against cancer and it has anti-estrogenic indoles. High-soluble fiber can also be found in broccoli which helps you to lose weight. Other great vegetables are kale, cauliflower, cabbage, and bok choy.

Spinach – This is an alkaline food that prevents bone and muscle loss. It can also protect you against cancer and heart diseases because it contains a lot of nutrients.

Turkey – Turkey only contains almost 0g of saturated fat this is even better than lesser than the most lean beef which has 4.5 g of saturated fat.

Quinoa – This is rich in fiber and protein and it is considered to be a super grain. It contains more fiber compared to oats and rice. You can eat this with spinach and meat.

Oats - This helps in reducing cholesterol, and it contains a lot of soluble fiber. You can add this to shakes you drink after your workout.

Tomatoes – It is known to have a high level of lycopene which helps fight against cancer. The lycopene that is in tomato paste is 4 times more than tomatoes that are fresh.

Oranges – This contains vitamin c that battles against diseases, magnesium for high blood pressure prevention, beta-carotene, and anti-oxidants. Do not drink the orange juice that is processed because it has a lot of sugar.

Apples – There is pectin in apples which helps with weight loss and next to cranberries, apples are contain the most anti-oxidants that comes from the peel. It is ideal to go organic when eating apples because they are highly contaminated by pesticides.

Carrots – They contain a lot of vitamin A which is very good for the eyes and they are high in fiber, low in calories, and they can be eaten even when raw because they taste good.

Green tea – This is a very good antioxidant and it is also a diuretic. It helps in making fat loss become faster, cancer prevention, and your blood circulation will improve. Drink this instead of coffee and it is always bets to drink the real ones and not the tea bags.

It is important that you do not consume plenty of carbohydrates and sugar because it will not be good for the overall formation of your muscles. It can even slow down your process of weight loss. Go for foods that are all-natural and rich in fiber and protein. It is also important that the food you eat does not contain a lot of chemicals. You should develop the habit of reading food labels, nutrition facts, and the ingredients before buying. You want to eat foods that do not have a long list of ingredients at the back especially if they are terms that you really do not understand. You can buy books that will tell you what these words mean and how they can affect your health. It does not mean that you do not eat foods that contain these, but anything in excess is bad. If you can afford to stay all-natural with your diet, it is best to do that.

Chapter 3. Strength Training Exercises

Squats overhead press

Stand straight with your feet hip-width apart with your elbows bent and hold 5 pounds of dumbbell in each hand keeping them at shoulder level. Your palms need to be facing forward. Start lowering into a squat and stretch your arms over your head while trying to stand up.

Do this for 3 reps with 15 repetitions.

Single-leg dumbbell row

Hold a 5 to 10 dumbbell in one hand and start hinging forward. Make sure that back is flat and you are parallel to the floor. Start extending your arm with the dumbbell towards the floor and your palm should be facing inside. Lift the opposite leg to the extended are to form a letter 'T'. Bend the arm holding the dumbbell until it is even with your torso. Stay in this position for a few seconds.

Do this for 15 repetitions on each arm for 3 sets.

Squat jumps

Stand straight with feet hip distance apart. Lower yourself to the ground until you feel your heels lifting, but maintain a flat back and look straight ahead. Pause and then jump with your legs fully extended and land soft on your feet. Your abdominals need to be engaged and your back flat until you finish the movement.

You can start by doing mini jumps for 10 to 15 reps.

Slow bicep curls

Stand straight with your feet hip width apart and with 5 pound dumbbells on each hand. Start to rotate both of your arms making the palms face forward. Start to bend your left arm on the elbows until your shoulders and hold this for 10 seconds before returning to former position. Do the same thing on your right hand.

Do this for 12 repetitions on each arm.

Stair climbing

Stand at the bottom of the stairs with both of your arms at your sides and your feet hip distance apart. Get in a push-up position that is about 4 to 5 steps up keeping your abdominals tight and get your torso rigid.

Put one hand on the next step and one hand to climb the next step and then get back down to where you started.

Walk for 15 times on each side.

How many days in a week should you strength train?

You need a very well-balanced amount of cardio and strength training to keep your body from hitting a plateau that can cause sudden stop of weight loss. You can do 3 to 4 days of cardiovascular workouts and 2 days of strength training. Adding a little variety to your workout such as this can your routine more variety and you will be able to train different muscle groups. Never workout 7 days in a week and you always need 1 day of rest to allow your muscles to rebuild and relax to have better results. When you are doing cardio exercises, give 30 to 40 minutes per workout session and for strength training, do not exceed 1 hour. You can do 30 to 45 minutes of strength training so that you will end up overtraining yourself. After 1 hour the muscle building hormones are no longer active so any exercise that you do beyond 1 hour is technically useless.

Chapter 4. Training Plan

For The Cardio

Workout 1

Do first a 5 to 10 minute general cardiovascular warm up exercise and then dynamic drills for 5 to 10 minutes of skipping and stretching exercises.

Get on a treadmill for 30 seconds running at the maximum incline. Put a mat, dumbbell, exercise ball, and ab wheel.

- Do a hill sprint for 30 seconds and get off, but keep it on

- Do an elbow plank for 30 seconds on the exercise ball

- Sprint again for 30 seconds

- Do 30 reverse crunches with dumbbells in both hands

- Sprint again for 30 seconds

- From your knees, do 30 ab wheel rollouts

Do this routine for 10 times.

Cool down for 10 minutes with a light cardio

Workout 2

Do first a 5 to 10 minute general cardiovascular warm up exercise and then dynamic drills for 5 to 10 minutes of skipping and stretching exercises.

Get on a treadmill and put it at maximum incline. Sprint for 60 seconds

- Do a 60 second sprint and get off, but keep it on

- Do kneeling ab crunches for 20 counts

- Get the heaviest dumbbells that you are capable of carrying and do a farmer's carry. Go and walk the farthest that you can and then return the dumbbells to the floor

- Do a 60 second sprint again

- Do medicine ball tosses on each side for 20 counts

- Do the farmer's carry again doing the same procedure as the previous one

Do the same routine for 6 to 8 times.

Finish off with a cool down of 5 to 10 minutes doing a cardiovascular workout

Workout

Week 1

Sunday – Rest

Monday – Do a full body workout of A

Tuesday – Do cardio workout 1

Wednesday – Do a full body workout of B

Thursday – Rest

Friday – Do a full body workout of A

Saturday – Do a cardio workout 2

Week 2

Sunday- Rest

Monday – Do a full body workout of B

Tuesday – Do a cardio workout 1

Wednesday – Do a full body workout of A

Thursday – Rest

Friday – Do a full body workout of B

Saturday – Do a cardio workout 2

Week 3

Sunday – Rest

Monday – Do a full body workout of A

Tuesday – Do a cardio workout 1

Wednesday – Do a full body workout of B

Thursday – Rest

Friday – Do a fully body workout of A

Saturday – Do a cardio workout 2

Week 4

Sunday – Rest

Monday – Do a full body workout of B

Tuesday – Do a cardio workout 1

Wednesday – Do a full body workout of A

Thursday – Rest

Friday – Do a full body workout of B

Saturday – Do a cardio workout 2

Week 5

Sunday – Rest

Monday – Do a full body workout of A

Tuesday – Do a cardio workout 1

Wednesday – Do a full body workout of B

Thursday – Rest

Friday – Do a fully body workout of A

Saturday – Do a cardio workout 2

Week 6

Sunday – Rest

Monday – Do a full body workout of B

Tuesday – Do a cardio workout 1

Wednesday – Do a full body workout of A

Thursday – Rest

Friday – Do a full body workout of B

Saturday – Do a cardio workout 2

Workout A: Full Body

A1 – Barbell Front Squat

For week 1

For 6 minutes, do 5 reps of 10 RM

For week 2

For 8 minutes, do 5 reps of 10 RM

For week 3

For 10 minutes, do 5 reps of 10 RM

For week 4

For 12 minutes, do 5 reps of 10 RM

For week 5

For 14 minutes, do 5 reps of 10 RM

For week 6

For 15 minutes, do 5 reps of 10 RM

A2 – Pull up

For week 1

For 6 minutes, do 5 reps

For week 2

For 8 minutes, do 5 reps

For week 3

For 10 minutes, do 5 reps

For week 4

For 12 minutes, do 5 reps

For week 5

For 14 minutes, do 5 reps

For week 6

For 15 minutes, do 5 reps

B1- Romanian Dead Lift

For week 1

For 6 minutes, do 5 reps of 10 RM

For week 2

For 8 minutes, do 5 reps of 10 RM

For week 3

For 10 minutes, do 5 reps of 10 RM

For week 4

For 12 minutes, do 5 reps of 10 RM

For week 5

For 14 minutes, do 5 reps of 10 RM

For week 6

For 15 minutes, do 5 reps of 10 RM

B2 – Dumbbell bench press using single arm

Week 1

For 6 minutes, Do 5 reps on left and right arm

Week 2

For 8 minutes, Do 5 reps on left and right arm

Week 3

For 10 minutes, Do 5 reps on left and right arm

Week 4

For 12 minutes, Do 5 reps on left and right arm

Week 5

For 14 minutes, Do 5 reps on left and right arm

Week 6

For 15 minutes, Do 5 reps on left and right arm

C – Barbell complex

For week 1

Do this exercise for 3 sets with 6 repetitions

For week 2

Do this exercise for 3 sets with 8 repetitions

For week 3

Do this exercise for 3 sets with 6 repetitions

For week 4

Do this exercise for 3 sets with 8 repetitions

For week 5

Do this exercise for 3 sets with 6 repetitions

For week 6

Do this exercise for 3 sets with 8 repetitions

D- Push-ups with a dumbbell

For week 1

Do 100 push-ups as fast as you can

For week 2

Do 100 push-ups as fast as you can

For week 3

Do 100 push-ups as fast as you can

For week 4

Do 100 push-ups as fast as you can

For week 5

Do 100 push-ups as fast as you can

For week 6

Do 100 push-ups as fast as you can

Workout B: Full Body

A1 – The conventional deadlift

For week 1

For 6 minutes, do 5 reps of 10 RM

For week 2

For 8 minutes, do 5 reps of 10 RM

For week 3

For 10 minutes, do 5 reps of 10 RM

For week 4

For 12 minutes, do 5 reps of 10 RM

For week 5

For 14 minutes, do 5 reps of 10 RM

For week 6

For 15 minutes, do 5 reps of 10 RM

A2 – Dumbbell row that is supported by the chest

For week 1

For 6 minutes, do 5 reps of 10 RM

For week 2

For 8 minutes, do 5 reps of 10 RM

For week 3

For 10 minutes, do 5 reps of 10 RM

For week 4

For 12 minutes, do 5 reps of 10 RM

For week 5

For 14 minutes, do 5 reps of 10 RM

For week 6

For 15 minutes, do 5 reps of 10 RM

B1 – Bulgarian Split Squat

For week 1

For 6 minutes, Do 5 reps on left and right arm

For week 2

For 8 minutes, Do 5 reps on left and right arm

For week 3

For 10 minutes, Do 5 reps on left and right arm

For week 4

For 12 minutes, Do 5 reps on left and right arm

For week 5

For 14 minutes, Do 5 reps on left and right arm

For week 6

For 15 minutes, Do 5 reps on left and right arm

B2 – Overhead press with a single arm

For week 1

For 6 minutes, Do 5 reps on left and right arm

For week 2

For 8 minutes, Do 5 reps on left and right arm

For week 3

For 10 minutes, Do 5 reps on left and right arm

For week 4

For 12 minutes, Do 5 reps on left and right arm

For week 5

For 14 minutes, Do 5 reps on left and right arm

For week 6

For 15 minutes, Do 5 reps on left and right arm

C- Barbell Complex

For week 1

Do this exercise for 3 sets with 6 repetitions

For week 2

Do this exercise for 3 sets with 8 repetitions

For week 3

Do this exercise for 3 sets with 6 repetitions

For week 4

Do this exercise for 3 sets with 8 repetitions

For week 5

Do this exercise for 3 sets with 6 repetitions

For week 6

Do this exercise for 3 sets with 8 repetitions

D- Suspension row that is inverted

For week 1

Do suspension row that is inverted for 100 times as fast as you can

For week 2

Do suspension row that is inverted for 100 times as fast as you can

For week 3

Do suspension row that is inverted for 100 times as fast as you can

For week 4

Do suspension row that is inverted for 100 times as fast as you can

For week 5

Do suspension row that is inverted for 100 times as fast as you can

For week 6

Do suspension row that is inverted for 100 times as fast as you can

Reminders

This is not an easy task and be sure to eat the right diet to support your weight loss and strength training. Enough sleep is also very important so be sure to get at least 7 hours of sleep every night because it will help your body recover faster from workouts and always stay hydrated. You can snack on healthy food when you feel hungry and stay away from sugar and a lot of saturated fat. Pack up on protein, iron, zinc, fiber, and calcium. If your diet is not good, you will not see the results that you want. Always count the calories that you are eating per day and make sure that you are not taking more than what is recommended. The 2 rest days are supposed to be maximized, but don't be totally sedentary as well. Do small errands in the house that will make you move because even if it's your rest day, staying on the couch the whole day is not healthy for your routine and health overall. It is also not a reason for you to have a "cheat day" because they really don't work and you can gain all the calories you've lost from the previous days. To avoid "cheat days", do not deprive yourself of everything and if you are craving for something, eat it but only take a bit or two and stop. Allowing yourself to eat foods that you like will prevent you from having cheat days. Read more about this tip when you search for the 80/20 rule in dieting.

Conclusion

The first thing you need to work on is yourself because without the determination and discipline, you will not the results that you want and deserve. No matter how much your workout, you will not see any difference if you do not stick to a good diet. You're only human so it's okay to give in to your cravings once in a while, but do not overindulge because it will all be useless. If you are strong and have a healthy body, you will gain self-esteem and self-confidence which are both important in living a better life. The benefits of losing weight and being strong do not stop with your body, but it will also have psychological effects on you too. Always remember that being at your best is your gift to the world and you can start by getting yourself healthier and fit. This is important if you have a family because you want to be there when they grow up and they want to see you strong even when you are already 50 or 70. Think about the happiness that it can bring you and the people around if you are healthy.

Thank You Page

I want to personally thank you for reading my book. I hope you found information in this book useful and I would be very grateful if you could leave your honest review about this book. I certainly want to thank you in advance for doing this.

If you have the time, you can check my other books too.

www.ingramcontent.com/pod-product-compliance
Lightning Source LLC
LaVergne TN
LVHW021744060526
838200LV00052B/3462